The Microbiome:
Leaky Gut Syndrome & Digestive Function

Raphael Kellman, MD

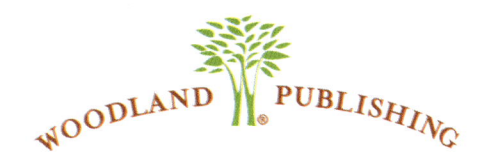

WOODLAND PUBLISHING

Copyright © 2019 by Raphael Kellman, MD

All rights reserved. No part of this publication may be reproduced, stored in a retrieval system, or transmitted in any form without the prior written permission of the copyright owner.

For permissions, ordering information, or bulk quantity discounts, contact:
Woodland Publishing, Salt Lake City, Utah
Visit our website: www.woodlandpublishing.com
Toll-free number: (800) 777-BOOK

The information in this book is for educational purposes only and is not recommended as a means of diagnosing or treating an illness. All matters concerning physical and mental health should be supervised by a health practitioner knowledgeable in treating that particular condition. Neither the publisher nor the author directly or indirectly dispenses medical advice, nor do they prescribe any remedies or assume any responsibility for those who choose to treat themselves.

Cataloging-in-Publication data is available from the Library of Congress.

ISBN: 978-1-58054-488-7

Printed in the United States of America

Contents

Intro	5
Microbiome 101	5
How Gastrointestinal Problems Arise	7
Leaky Gut And Gastrointestinal Concerns	10
Functional Medicine Testing	11
The Microbiome Protocol	12
Probiotics	21
Which Probiotics Are Right For Me?	23
Bacteria Strains	25
Microbiome Superfoods	29
Notes	32
About the Author	33

Intro

Are you one of the 70,000,000 people plagued by debilitating digestive disorders—irritable bowel syndrome, leaky gut, constipation, diarrhea, acid reflux, GERD and SIBO, Crohn's Disease, or even the mildest form of upset stomach? (NOTE #1)

Why do so many people have these issues? Without question, the reasons are many—and complicated. A lot of blame can be placed on our love affair with processed foods and fast foods. The typical American diet lacks whole, fresh, chemical and process-free foods. (NOTE #2) Other culprits lurk in every pharmacy in America. Antacids, laxatives, stool softeners—while not terrible as an occasional remedy—can cause tremendous havoc on our systems over time. Our bodies are designed to eat whole foods, retain essential nutrients for energy and fuel, and eliminate waste. Our overconsumption of processed foods, sugar, artificial and fast food disrupts that basic flow, and these fast-fix "remedies" actually worsen the problems. Even more severe are the Proton Pump Inhibitors (PPI's) which—when taken for a long period of time—can completely throw your system out of whack for many years. PPI's inhibit the body from producing stomach acid. However, some of that acid is essential for proper digestion, and to absorb calcium and other nutrients. Add to that our sedentary, stressful lifestyles, and it's easy to see why millions suffer from some sort of GI concerns.

Although the symptoms, diagnoses, and reasons are many, we have some very good news for you. In the vast majority of cases, there's a reason for it. At my functional medicine practice in New York City, virtually ALL of my patients experience some type of gastrointestinal tract issue at one point or another. Why is that? What does it mean? And what easy steps can you do TODAY to take matters in your own hands and feel good again? We're going to explore all of that (and more) in this book.

Microbiome 101

I bet you've been hearing the word "microbiome" being tossed around lately. It's become one of those hot buzzwords in science, in diets, and in medicine. It's been written about in all of the women's magazines—even Time Magazine and the Wall Street Journal have written articles about this microbiome. But what exactly is it? And more important, what role does it play in your health? To put it briefly, we are made up of bacteria. In fact, life would not be possible without bacteria. Bacteria significantly outnumber our genes. (NOTE #3) And these bacteria are quite brilliant. They can transfer DNA to each other, they can self-mutate and respond to their environment. They communicate to each other. (NOTE #4)

They have all the elements of conscious life.

- Bacteria were the first life forms to exist on Earth
- They are responsible for carbon and nitrogen cycles; without which there would be no life
- They developed photosynthesis
- They created the Earth's atmospheric oxygen
- They inhabit every environment on Earth
- They are greater in mass than all the fish in the sea and animals on the land
- The amount of DNA that they contain and exchange is incomprehensible.

In fact, bacteria are everywhere!

- Air, water, soil, animals, people, food, plants, ocean, core of the earth
- Cheese, yogurt, other dairy products
- Certain medicines
- Inside your intestines, teeth

Bacteria are the sine qua non of life; they contain the software of healing. Only when we add the right strains to our diet can we begin to really heal at the deepest level.

I see thousands and thousands of sick patients at my practice. If there is one common element to all disease, is that almost all diseases have some element of microbiome dysfunction. Whether there be an anxiety issue, insomnia, autoimmune, cognitive or digestive/gastrointestinal issue (or, in a large percent of cases, a combination of many symptoms), I always start by looking at the gut. And, invariably, that is where we find an imbalance. When the microbiome is functioning optimally, the body leans to optimal functioning. When we heal the microbiome, we are able to heal not only the issue that the patient first presented, but that "vitality" or zest for life also returns. We are able to pinpoint exactly what supplements and dietary changes are needed through conversation, history and testing. This precise targeting of bacterial imbalance is what I call "MICROBIOME MEDICINE." And the very good news is that with today's targeted probiotics now available, with a little bit of research and knowledge, you can actually take your health matters into your own hands. Wonderful news!

How Gastrointestinal Problems Arise

For way too long, bacteria were positioned as our enemies. An industry of anti-bacterial super-hygiene products was born. The world became over-sterilized—even children who were once allowed and encouraged to play in the dirt, are now told that soil is bad. Simultaneously, the toxins we are exposed to in our environment are expanding. Personal skincare products, processed food, household cleaning products, air pollution, water contamination—all laden with toxic substances, which seeps into our bloodstream.

Eventually these chemicals become part of our bodies' container system. As these chemicals are recognized as foreign aliens by the body, the immune system reacts with inflammation. And inflammation is the root of virtually all disease. (NOTE #5)

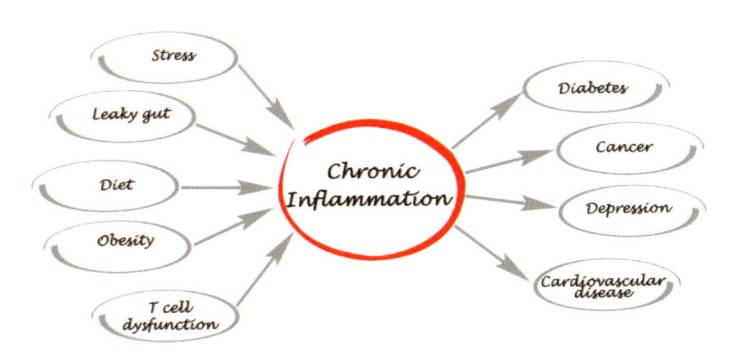

Are you aware that most of your immune system—seventy five percent—is inside the gut wall? Therefore, inflammation, which can damage the gut wall (which is more and more common) causes more inflammation and autoimmune response. The gut wall is our protection against pathogens. Therefore, retaining its integrity is the most significant defense against disease. Practically every aspect of the body is affected by the health of the microbiome.

The microbiome is like your body's control center. It produces vitamins, absorbs nutrients, and generates neurotransmitters like those produced by your brain. An optimal microbiome is balanced with a diverse range of bacteria and in the right ratio. As long as we are able to keep the microbiome healthy, chances are that we will remain healthy. And it's the reason why so many of us experience brain fog, fatigue and other symptoms when we have digestive and leaky gut issues.

In an optimal microbiome, the walls of the intestine are strong, which translates into a strong immune response. It heals itself as it introduces nutrients that maintain a healthy gut wall. However, maintaining a strong gut wall is difficult for even the most aware. If you currently avoid preservatives, processed foods, pesticides, antibiotics, antibiotic-fed poultry, you're definitely on the right track, but chances are very high that there is still a toxic residue in your gut. If you use proton pump inhibitors, take NSAID's, or are under chronic stress, your risk for a compromised microbiome is unfortunately, greater.

When unhealthy substances are ingested, over time the gut wall will begin to lose its integrity. The wall becomes porous, with the emergence of small holes resembling a fine mesh. When there is leaky gut, toxins and unwanted bacteria can seep through and induce inflammation, which can cause systemic damage.

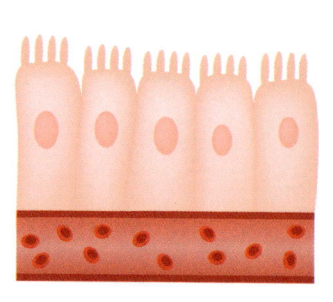

Normal Tight Junction   **Leaky and Inflamed**

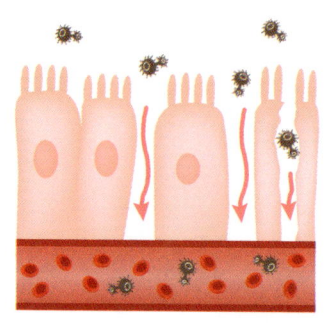

The bacterial ecology is a powerful lifeforce.

Many factors may upset the GI tract and its motility (ability to keep moving), including:

- Eating a diet low in fiber
- Not enough exercise
- Eating large amounts of dairy products
- Stress
- Resisting the urge to have a bowel movement
- Resisting the urge to have bowel movements due to pain from hemorrhoids
- Overusing laxatives (stool softeners) that, over time, weaken the bowel muscles
- Antacid medicines
- Certain medicines (especially antidepressants, iron pills, narcotics)

Leaky Gut first presents itself as distressing gastrointestinal tract issues—bloating, pain, constipation and diarrhea. Individuals start to accept these symptoms as part of everyday life, or they take drugstore remedies to mask the symptoms. Of course, most are unaware that these medications are causing more and more damage to that already weakened gut. We can mask the symptoms for a while, but we can only really heal—at the deepest level—when we take a deeper look into the root causes, and not just the symptoms

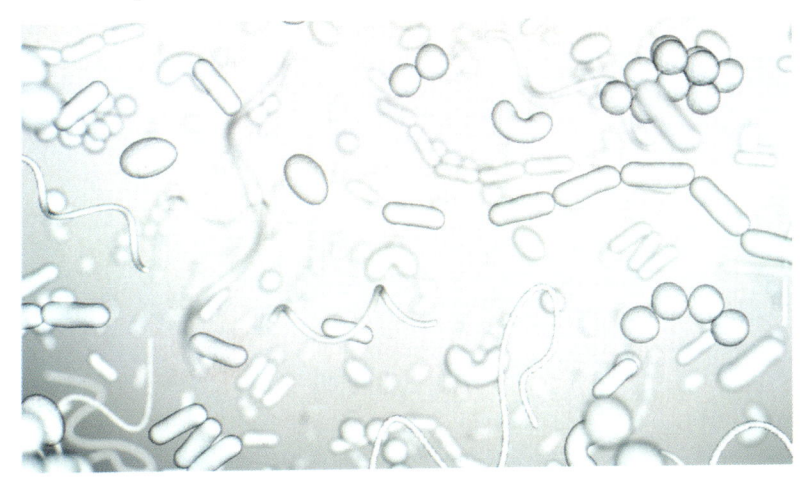

Leaky Gut And Gastrointestinal Concerns

In a leaky gut, the tight junctions working like a glue meant to hold the outer layers of intestinal cells tightly together start to loosen. The mucosal layer surrounding the gut wall weakens. Food particles and even bacteria escape into the bloodstream. Since the immune system is on the other side of the gut wall, the partially digested food/and or bacteria initiate an immune response in the form of inflammation. With repetitive assaults, the immune system goes into overdrive and can start attacking healthy tissue.

Why is this so dangerous?

The gut bacteria are the repository for your DNA. Every twenty seconds, the microorganisms reproduce themselves. And along with it they replicate the changes that have happened to them as a result of an altered bacterial environment. The genetic code (your unique genome) that was present at birth may be affected.

The leaky gut creates an imbalance in the microbiome. The imbalanced microbiome responds with more dysfunction which may even extend outside the gut. For instance, since the gut and the brain are in communication, problems may show up as impaired cognition, poor memory and depression. Once we can reverse this vicious circle by removing toxins, replenishing with prebiotic and probiotic foods and proper, targeted probiotics, the pathway to healing can be established.

Irritable Bowel Syndrome, GERD, acid reflux, constipation—virtually ALL gastrointestinal disorders come as a result of a sparse microbiome that is devoid of the rich, varied species known to confer health benefits. Once the ecology is thrown off, holes and empty pockets allow for more opportunistic and virulent strains to colonize and multiply over time. In this environment, without proper treatment to restore the gut microbiome to a vibrant and diverse state, patients suffer a wide range of conditions. Affecting areas as far away as the brain, it can spark mood disorders, as well as declines in cognition. Autoimmunity often ensues, including the possibility for Type 2 diabetes, and as the immune system suffers, IBS and IBD become more likely.

Functional Medicine Testing

When treating patients with gastrointestinal concerns, my first step is to study the function of the entire body and microbiome. We start with comprehensive testing that goes well beyond the standard. DNA stool analysis gives an in-depth understanding of pathogens such as parasites, yeast, opportunistic bacterial populations, inflammation and the way the intestinal immune system is functioning. An ion test uses blood and urine to measure the way the body is absorbing and using nutrients, making energy, and also measures metabolites produced by different bacteria in the intestine. Comprehensive blood testing might be performed to uncover hidden issues such as undiagnosed low thyroid, which is frequently present in patients who suffer from gastrointestinal disorders. The highly specialized **TRH stimulation test** is often necessary, simply because highly inflammatory conditions suppress TSH in the body, rendering the routine thyroid test ineffective. This is key, since the intestine is exquisitely dependent on thyroid hormone in order to function. In my opinion, the TRH stimulation test is one of the most important tools in our toolbox—and one that unfortunately many practitioners (even functional medicine doctors) are not offering. If you have any thyroid-based concerns—even if your doctor has told you your numbers are "normal" but you know something is still not right, I urge you to dig deeper to find someone who administers this test.

> *But, even if you don't have access to these tests, do not despair! There are many things one can do on their own to greatly improve their microbiome and regain gastrointestinal balance.*

The cornerstone for virtually all illnesses—as well as to maintain good health—starts with what I call the FOUR R's. Following this regimen will set the stage for you to heal your own ailments, and set you on a course of good health, focus and vitality. The 4R program works to restore and improve healthy bacterial populations without further damaging the ecology—often the result of continued antibiotic use. (Note: not all of our antibiotic intake comes from medicine. The poultry we eat also contains large amounts of antibiotics. (NOTE #6) I urge you to consider consuming only organic, grass fed meat and poultry as an important step in regaining your health and vitality.)

The Microbiome Protocol
The Four R's:

| REMOVE | REINOCULATE |
| REPLACE | REPAIR |

1. REMOVE the Foods That Disrupt Your Whole Ecology

A proper ecology is about balance: a healthy exchange among all the different elements of the system. Load up on the foods that will support your microbiome and your gut. And it's equally as important to avoid those foods that disrupt your ecology.

This is especially important if you struggle with leaky gut, which is when a permeable intestinal wall allows partially digested foods and toxins to pass through the gut into the immune system, where it triggers an inflammatory response. Enough inflammatory responses and you develop a food sensitivity, where inflammation is triggered every time you consume even the smallest particle of a particular food. Develop enough food sensitivities and your whole body is suffused with chronic inflammation, a continually burning flame that promotes a number of health conditions, including anxiety, depression, and brain fog.

Think of this diet as a medical prescription that is helping your system heal. After you've spent at least three weeks on this protocol, it is possible to slowly add a small amount of these items into your diet. But for now, please, avoid all of the following foods. Your gastrointestinal tract and your immune system need to rest in order to heal.

What To Avoid:

Processed or packaged foods

Soy
(exceptions are soy lecithin and organic fermented soy: soy sauce, tempeh and miso)

Soy protein isolate
which is found in many protein bars, protein shakes and protein powders.

Sugars and sweeteners
natural or artificial, except monk fruit

Trans fats and hydrogenated fats

Canola and Cottonseed Oil
These oils are highly processed, genetically modified, and full of chemicals. Canola oil may also pose dangers to the myelin sheath that coats your nerves, triggering a number of disturbing symptoms.

Corn and Cornstarch
Since the vast majority of the U.S. corn crop has been genetically modified, I'd prefer you to avoid corn products to protect both your microbiome and your overall health. Besides, corn is a sweet, starchy grain that can overfeed certain bacteria, helping to unbalance your microbiome.

Cow's Milk Dairy Products
Cow's milk dairy products are some of the most likely to trigger an inflammatory reaction. They are difficult for many people to digest, and I've noticed that virtually everyone with leaky gut has a cow's milk dairy sensitivity. Sadly, conventionally farmed dairy products are loaded with hormones, which disrupt *your* hormones, and with antibiotics, which further disrupt your microbiome.

Dried or Canned Fruits, Fruit Juice
(loaded with sugar)

Gluten
Even non-Celiac individuals can have gluten sensitivities. Many people find gluten-bearing grains difficult to digest, which sets you up for gut problems. Gluten also creates zonulin, a protein that opens the tight junctions in your intestinal wall, helping to create leaky gut, which in turn produces brain fog and many other types of brain dysfunction.

High Fructose Corn Syrup

Iceberg Lettuce
Toxic insecticides disrupt your gut, your microbiome, and your endocrine system—so, please stay away from this least nutritious of all the lettuces and opt for highly nutritious organic dark leafy greens instead.

Peanuts or Peanut Butter
Opt for healthier legumes. Peanuts frequently contain aflotoxin, a toxin found in various molds.

Processed Foods, Meats and Deli Meats
Loaded with gluten, unhealthy fats, sugar, high fructose corn syrup, and nitrates, processed foods and meats are a quadruple threat to your gut and microbiome, and can even be carcinogenic. In addition, I urge you to consume only organic chicken to avoid pesticides and antibiotics.

Please stay away from these foods for a minimum of three weeks. If you've been having leaky gut, digestive issues or other gastrointestinal distress, and anxiety, depression, brain fog or fatigue, it would probably be beneficial to take a three-month break from cow's milk. After that, it might be possible to slowly re-introduce it into your diet sparingly, cutting back or avoiding it entirely at the first sign of symptoms. In fact, once your gastrointestinal tract is healthy, it is entirely possible to enjoy whatever you want in moderation.

People with autoimmune issues or leaky gut frequently have parasites or yeast. (NOTE #7) Therefore, we supplement with natural products that will destroy them:

Berberine—one of the most versatile and effective natural supplements available. It lowers blood sugar, improves gut function, and improves heart health, to name a few. It works at the cellular level and, much like a pharmaceutical, has the capacity to change the cells' function. It activates AMPK, an enzyme known to regulate metabolism (NOTE #8)

Wormwood
Caprylic acid
Grapefruit seed extract—look for natural GFSE without synthetic contaminants.
Garlic
Oregano Oil
Olive Leaf Extract
Black Seed Oil—look for nigella sativa, not black cumin seed oil.

At the end of this initial phase, inflammation will begin to lessen, fat-burning will become more efficient, and your overall sense of wellness might even start to return.

2. REPLACE the digestive enzymes that you need for optimal digestion.

Now that we've removed the disruptors, we can work on adding the important building blocks to rebuild your microbiome for optimal bacterial balance. If you suffer from gastrointestinal issues, particularly acid reflux (quite common among all digestive concerns)—then you've probably have had your share of over-the-counter and prescription antacids. But the truth is that most Americans suffer from *too little* stomach acid, not too much. In fact, the most common reason for heartburn (acid reflux) is not having *enough* stomach acid to properly break down proteins. Undigested food hangs around in your stomach along with the insufficient acid—and then, sometimes finds its way back into the esophagus, where the acid burns.

We need adequate enzymes and stomach acids in order to digest our food. Low stomach acid is a major player in the development of leaky gut. By adding it back into your routine, you will then be able to absorb those much-needed nutrients. With every meal or snack take one of the following:

Raw Apple Cider Vinegar–ACV is rich in enzymes that can break down bacteria in food. Raw apple cider vinegar is also effective in reducing symptoms from acid reflux, diabetes, and high blood sugar. (Note: Don't drink it straight up as it can damage your teeth. Dilute one teaspoon in ¼ cup of water and drink it before each meal. You can also look for ACV capsules or tablets that deliver the acetic acid in the stomach.

Ginger–This ancient herb is widely known for its anti-inflammatory properties, an alternative treatment for acid reflux and other gastrointestinal disorders.

500 mg Hydrochloric Acid tablet–at each meal, gradually increasing to 1000 mg. (This has the same effect as ACV.)

Over-the-Counter Digestive Enzymes–Take one at the beginning of each meal. There are many excellent choices available. Look for products containing the following ingredients:

- Protease, which digests protein
- Lipase, which digests fat
- Amylase, which digests carbohydrates including starches
- DPP IV, which helps digest gluten and casein (milk protein)
- Alpha-galactosidase: breaks down carbohydrates, complex sugars and fat

And, to improve digestion, brain function, and gut function, I highly recommend:
Butyrate or Beta-Hydroxybutyrate (BHB): 2 pills, 2 times a day (not only a superstar in improving digestion, butyrate improves brain function as well)

NOTE: I can't say enough about the benefits of the powerhouse supplement Butyrate in treating many health conditions, especially Irritable Bowel Syndrome. Butyric acid belongs to a group of short-chain fatty acids and is thought to play several beneficial roles in the gastrointestinal tract. It is easily absorbed by cells and used as a main source of energy. Butyric acid is an important regulator of gastrointestinal tract motility. (NOTE #9)

3. RE-INOCULATE with prebiotics and targeted probiotics.

Our goal is to support an ideal balance of stomach acid. First step is to wean off of those antacids! (Note: If you're taking a Proton Pump Inhibitor, please wean under your doctor's guidance.) Then, we introduce prebiotics.

If you're asking yourself "What's the difference between probiotics and prebiotics?" don't worry—you're not alone! Here's my quick breakdown:

> *Probiotics* are microscopic organisms that replenish your microbiome, or bacterial ecology. *Prebiotics* are foods and supplements that nourish the organisms already in your microbiome.

And, to answer your next question—in order to have a balanced microbiome and begin the healing process to finally feel free of your digestive disorders, acid reflux, weak metabolism, leaky gut, constipation, diarrhea, etc., you need **both** Probiotics *and* Prebiotics. They work hand in hand; together they can make a significant improvement in your health.

> Our gut health, gastrointestinal tract balance, and metabolism depend on the balance of microbial balance within our gastrointestinal tract.

FUNCTIONS OF PREBIOTICS

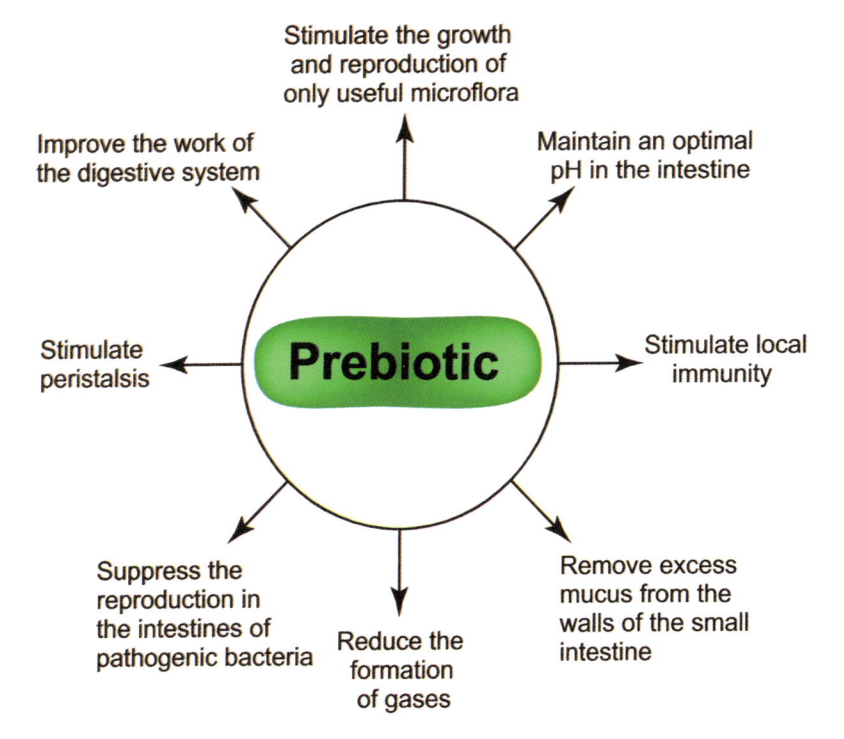

- Stimulate the growth and reproduction of only useful microflora
- Improve the work of the digestive system
- Maintain an optimal pH in the intestine
- Stimulate peristalsis
- Stimulate local immunity
- Suppress the reproduction in the intestines of pathogenic bacteria
- Reduce the formation of gases
- Remove excess mucus from the walls of the small intestine

Prebiotics are foods that nourish the bacteria in your bacterial ecology. They can be food or pill. Prebiotics are often referred to as fertilizer because they help your healthy bacteria flourish. In the case of plant foods, for example, they break down the fibers into digestible components.

Luckily, prebiotics are very easy to add to your diet. Here are some of the top "microbiome superfoods." (In the back of this book is a longer Microbiome Superfood and Spice checklist.)

Jerusalem Artichokes (also called "Sunchokes")
Asparagus
Carrots
Garlic
Jicama
Leeks
Onions
Radishes

Fermented foods: Yogurt, Kefir, Miso, Kombucha, Sauerkraut, Pickles (Fermented vegetables are also associated with strengthening immune function, promoting weight loss, and lowering blood pressure.)

In addition to these superfoods, it is essential to add plant fiber to your diet to nourish and feed your microbiome. There are three types of natural high fiber foods that will benefit your microbiome—and your overall health: arabinogalactans, inulin, and resistant starches. Add a few from each category, consume raw whenever possible, and please purchase organic whenever you can.

Arabinogalactans

Arabinogalactans feed your lactobacillus and bifidobacterium, two types of bacteria that are crucial to your microbial community. This type of fiber is essential in repairing a leaky gut. Arabinogalactans ferment in your intestinal tract, producing the short-chain fatty acids (SCFAs) that are essential to a healthy gut wall. These acids are used by the cells of your gut wall to produce energy, keeping your gut wall strong and vibrant. They also turn on your anti-inflammatory genes while turning off inflammatory genes, thus protecting your gut wall from inflammation, leaky gut, and gastrointestinal distress.

Foods rich in arabinogalactans include:

Carrots
Kiwi
Radishes
Tomatoes

Turmeric (look for Fermented Turmeric Root or Turmeric Root Extract 300 mg)
Pears
Larch Tree Bark (an excellent supplement for leaky gut sufferers)

Inulin

Your microbiome loves inulin! This type of natural fiber nourishes a wide variety of bacteria and is essential in maintaining gut and gastrointestinal health. Inulin is key to diversity as it feeds many different bacterial types. Inulin heals the gut and supports efficient digestion. Remember, consuming a nutrient isn't enough—your body has to *absorb* that nutrient in order to benefit. Many of my patients overdo the vitamins, hoping to boost their nutrition. But if your gut isn't properly absorbing nutrients, you're not getting any benefit from them. That's one important reason why you need to heal your gut, so that your body is able to absorb vitamins efficiently.

Foods rich in inulin include:

- Dandelion Greens
- Chicory Root
- Asparagus
- Barley
- Oats
- Apples
- Flax Seeds
- Onions
- Jerusalem Artichokes
- Bananas
- Wheat Bran
- Seaweed

Resistant Starches

You can find this type of plant fiber in the following foods:

Grains and pseudo-grains: millet, quinoa, rice
Legumes: beans of all types, garbanzos, lentils
Nuts: almonds, brazil nuts, chestnuts, hazelnuts, macadamia nuts, pecans, pine nuts, walnuts, nut butters and nut flours
Seeds: chia seeds, flaxseeds, pumpkin seeds, sesame seeds, sunflower seeds

Like arabinogalactans and inulin, resistant starches are indigestible—by *you*. Your microbiome, on the other hand, feeds on them quite happily, to the benefit of your gut. Resistant starches help your gut bacteria produce short-chain fatty acids, particularly the one known as *butyrate*. It's hard for me to praise butyrate too highly: it supports the cells that line your large intestine, helps regulate your metabolism, and lowers inflammation, which, as we have seen, is essential in treating virtually all disease.

4. REPAIR and Maintain a Healthy Gut.

In addition to prebiotics and probiotics, which nourish and feed the beneficial bacteria, certain supplements and healing foods do wonders to repair—and maintain—our gut function. Virtually all of our gastrointestinal and leaky gut patients are put on a regimen of some of these herbs and supplements along with their probiotics.

- L. Glutamine
- Quercetin
- Zinc
- N-acetyl Glucosamine
- DGL (a form of licorice)
- Slippery Elm
- Marshmallow
- Gamma Oryzni

REPAIR inflammation lining by taking L-Butyrate, a powerful anti-inflammatory and the herb Turmeric with Curcumin.
REPAIR the gut strength with L-Glutamine and minerals like Zinc.
REPAIR by restoring gut balance with the correct ratio of Omega 3 to Omega 6 by adding:

- Omega 3 dietary supplement
- Almonds
- Macadamia nuts
- Cashews
- Seeds and seed butters
- Flaxseed and flaxseed oil
- Olive oil

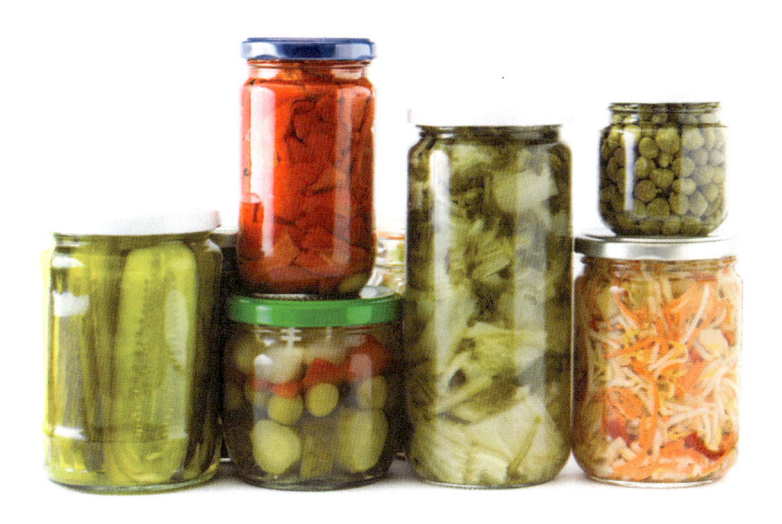

Probiotics

Now we've come to the crux of the matter. These amazing bacteria—when taken in the right form and with the right combination of strains—can do more to help you than any pharmaceutical product. Healing the gut leads to true healing *at the very deepest level*, and targeted probiotics are truly the new frontier in medicine. They act like natural antibiotics and add vitamins and proteins that seal the gut wall, reduce inflammation, enhance the immune system, speed metabolism, balance blood sugar, fight depression and anxiety, and even reverse cognitive decline. (NOTE #10)

No pharmaceutical can be compared to probiotics.

Probiotics To Maintain The Gut Barrier

Probiotics help maintain gut health in many ways:

1. Promoting mucous secretion. Our intestinal wall includes a mucous layer that wards off inhospitable microbes. Probiotics can increase the production of mucin, the slimy substance that coats and protects this layer.

2. Many probiotic bacteria can produce antimicrobial substances that kill bad bacteria trying to make their way through the gut.

3. Lowering pH levels. Some probiotic strains produce lactic or acetic acid, which can make invader microbes like E-coli less likely to thrive by creating a more acidic gut environment.

4. Competing for binding sites on epithelial cells. When probiotics are in good supply, they can crowd out bad guy bacteria by taking over any available binding sites on cells and the mucous layer. Much like a crowded parking lot without any available spaces, the inhospitable bacteria can't settle in.

5. Increasing antibody levels. Probiotics can both increase levels of cells that produce antibodies (called immunoglobulins) and promote secretion of the antibodies—like sIgA—in the mucous layer.

6. Strengthening the structure of tight junctions. Beneficial bacteria help jump-start the assembly of tight junction proteins, and they activate cell-signaling that strengthens tight junctions so the bad guys can't push their way through.

In the next section of this book ("Which Probiotics?"), we're going to dig a little deeper and talk about which *specific* strains of bacteria work wonders on leaky gut, digestive issues, metabolism, constipation, irritable bowel, and more.

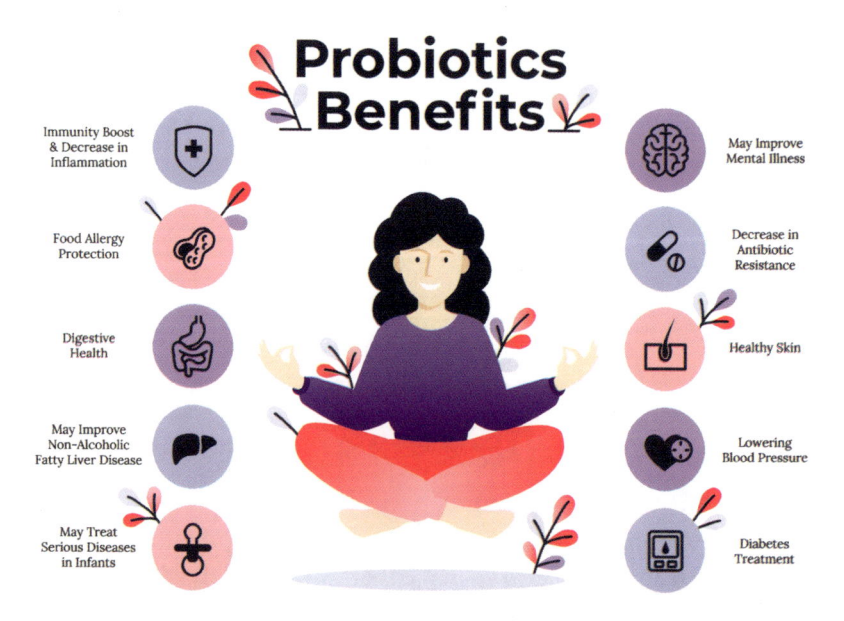

Probiotics Benefits

- Immunity Boost & Decrease in Inflammation
- Food Allergy Protection
- Digestive Health
- May Improve Non-Alcoholic Fatty Liver Disease
- May Treat Serious Diseases in Infants
- May Improve Mental Illness
- Decrease in Antibiotic Resistance
- Healthy Skin
- Lowering Blood Pressure
- Diabetes Treatment

Which Probiotics Are Right For Me?

This is where it gets exciting. We know what to eliminate and we know we need to repair our depleted microbiome with certain bacteria to regain healthy balance, or "ecology" as I like to call it. So now we look to the probiotics. And therein lie the answers. But as you've probably seen—hundreds of formulas now line the shelves of every health food store, pharmacy and supermarket. Which bacteria strains do you need? That my friends, is the question!

Before we get into which strains are beneficial for gastrointestinal concerns, let's talk for a moment about probiotics in general. By now you can certainly see the importance of adding probiotic supplements to your routine. But before you run out to your favorite natural foods store, let's just review certain criteria about your choice. Seems like every vitamin company is now jumping in on the probiotic trend and the choices can be dizzying. Luckily, I've spent a lot of time studying the efficacies, safety, shelf life and other probiotic attributes—and can help save you a lot of time examining all of those products!

1. Millions, Billions—and Trillions??

As a general rule, a probiotic should provide at least 1 billion CFUs (colony forming units, i.e., viable cells) per strain, with doses starting at 1 billion and ranging 10 billion to 50 billion or higher CFUs daily for adults.

When it comes to bacteria, it is truly the more the merrier.

2. Variety of strains

Within those billions of strains in a probiotic supplement, we want to see a wide variety of bacteria strains. As you're about to learn when we get into which strains I recommend to my leaky gut and gastrointestinal patients, these bacteria work in concert with each other. Having one but not certain others would be like going to a symphony without the strings section. Still music, but not nearly as effective.

3. Refrigeration

As you've probably noticed, most probiotics are in the supplement aisle of your store. But, some are tucked away in that small refrigerated section. Why is that? And what happens if you purchase them but then they sit in your car for most of the day—or even overnight?

For many probiotics, refrigeration is critical, as many probiotic bacteria are naturally sensitive to heat and moisture. Reputable manufacturers conduct stability tests to know how their probiotics perform in all conditions, especially when exposed to heat, moisture and stomach acid. We recommend you store them in your refrigerator to maintain maximum potency. Be careful about purchasing probiotics online as many companies do not cold store their probiotics.

4. Testing

Here's where I can save you hundreds (maybe thousands!) of dollars. I've actually seen the research—what manufacturers claim vs. what is actually entering your system and the variations are astonishing.

When selecting a probiotic, please do a little legwork—find out if the company making it can prove its efficacy. There are many, many expensive supplements out that there just aren't delivering. We want to make sure you find one that is delivering those powerful bacteria into your system. In our office in New York, we recommend probiotics from three or four manufacturers, depending on the patient's health criteria—and each of these makers have undergone rigorous testing to ensure efficacy and potency. If you would like a list of the specific brands we recommend, email us at info@kellmancenter.com. (Of course we cannot give medical advice without a medical examination but we can share the list of probiotics that we trust and recommend.)

Enteric Coating

There's a phrase you've probably seen on aspirin—but what exactly does it mean, and why exactly do you need it? I tell my patients that this is essential with probiotics (and aspirin for that matter). Enteric coating means that the product will survive your stomach acid and make its way into your small intestine, where it can begin to colonize and then travel throughout your body to do its job for maximum effectiveness. Also, look for natural enteric coatings, such as shellac, resin and other natural coatings. Avoid acrylics and other synthetic coatings which can damage the microbiome and disrupt the endocrine system.

Bacteria Strains

Now onto the fun stuff! Which bacteria are the ones that work for leaky gut? For bloating? Gas? Constipation? Irritable bowel? That's the magic! Figuring out which probiotics you need, which ones will put your system in balance. And, trust me, when you find that combination, you'll be amazed. Not only will your gastro concerns start to heal, but so will your energy, your mood, your zest for life!

Following are the specific bacterial strains that are proven to improve gastrointestinal dysfunction:

L. Plantarum

- Originates from human digestive tract
- Used to ferment foods like kimchi & sauerkraut
- Supports intestinal distress & gut permeability
- Reputed to crowd out gram-negative pathogenic bacteria by producing *bacteriocins*
- May provide allergy support by regulating mast cells and breaking down histamine
- Improves digestion, immunity, overall health
- Balances bacteria in the microbiome
- Research has shown significant improvement in IBS (95% saw huge improvement in all IBS symptoms vs. 5% on placebo)
- Helpful with gas, immune system and decreasing inflammatory response.
- Produces B vitamins and help with iron absorption
- Protects against heavy metal and reduce oxidative stress
- Increases dopamine and seratonin levels

L. Paracasei

- Supports respiratory & immune wellness through the production of *biosurfactants* that inhibit bacterial adhesion
- Supports the immune system through regulation of T-helper cells (Th1 & Th2)
- Helps balance gut bacteria, immune system, and improve the hyperimmune state.
- May provide mycotoxin support by inhibiting zearalenone (ZEN), an estrogenic mycotoxin found in most grains & cereals

B. Lactis (Animalis subsp. Lactis)

- Supports the digestion of sugars, especially lactose1
- Adheres easily to the intestinal wall, which may inhibit the ability for pathogenic bacteria to adhere to the wall of the intestines and colon
- Protects the intestines from zinc deficiency; zinc is important for the formation of biomembranes (plasma membrane of epithelial cells); zinc deficiency can lead to increased gut permeability & may also cause diarrhea
- Highly prevalent bacteria in the intestines & the colon
- Enhances immunity, fights tumor growth, improves digestion and can lower cholesterol
- Breaks down body waste
- Aids in the absorption of various vitamins and minerals
- Improves leaky gut along with other GI problems such as IBS symptoms, acute diarrhea and the converse, constipation
- Lessens the severity of respiratory infections, colds and the flu and on the skin
- Reduces allergic responses and accompanying inflammation
- Enhances the body's immune capability

B. Longum

- May support blood sugar health by improving metabolic rhythms involving glucose utilization
- May be beneficial to people with Celiac disease and/or gluten-intolerance, shown to lower immune response to gliadin, a gluten protein
- B. Longum may benefit people with fructose malabsorption (FODMAP, SIBO) as B. longum utilizes excess fructose as a food source

L. Rhamnosus

- Regulation of insulin, leptin (satiety hormone) & ghrelin (hunger hormone)

- Increases circulating leptin concentrations, supporting appetite management
- Supports cellular energy production through enzyme AMPK activation; AMPK is the "master metabolic regulator" that influences how cells process energy
- Research has shown that L. Rhamnosus helps with depression and executive function

L. Helveticus

- Lactobicillus Helveticus is a lactic acid bacteria. It's naturally found in the gut and in the urino-genital track.
- Improves gut health, treats gut infections
- Helps with blood pressure, anxiety and depression
- Improves sleep
- Supports serum calcium in the blood by absorbing calcium from the intestines, which may provide support for strong & healthy bones
- May provide support for mood, anxiety & depression by creating the neurotransmitters GABA, serotonin, catecholamines & acetylcholine
- Removes allergens from certain foods

S. Thermophilus

- May provide support for IBS & Crohn's through regulation of several inflammatory markers: IL-4, IL-5, IL-6, IL-10
- Supports athletic performance and recovery; clinical trials measured muscle strength, muscle soreness, muscle range of motion and muscle girth pre & post supplementation
- Helps maintain muscle strength & range of motion through regulation of IL-6 and CK inflammatory markers

B. Bifidum

- Converts Vitamin K into the active form your body can use
- Support for hair loss through K2 production
- Supports normal, healthy cholesterol levels by converting cholesterol into coprostanol so it can be excreted

L. Lactis

- Benefits the immune system
- May combat allergies and hypertension
- Has beneficial effects on the skin
- L. lactis has been the subject of a large amount of research for its usefulness as a vaccine vehicle

E. Faecum (Enterococcus Faecum)

- Enterococcus colonies typically found in the gastrointestinal tract
- Produces ATP, a compound which provides energy to the cells
- anti-microbial benefits
- E. Faecum indicated strong anti-viral activity against the food borne pathogens

L. Acidophilus

- Found in the intestines and vagina
- Present in fermented foods like sauerkraut, miso, tempeh
- L.acidophilus has been used to treat or prevent a wide range of ailments, including yeast infections, diarrhea, irritable bowel syndrome, lactose intolerance, intestinal problems, and urinary tract infections
- Performs better than yogurt in lowering LDL cholesterol

L.gasseri

- Known for its weight-reduction, obesity and metabolic syndrome properties
- Boosts immunity
- Helps with allergies
- Lowers cholesterol in combination with inulin

Microbiome Superfoods

Animal Proteins (Organic And Grass-Fed)

- Beef
- Chicken
- Lamb
- Venison
- Low-Mercury Fish
- Wild-Caught Salmon
- Shellfish
- Goat's Milk Dairy
- Sheep's Milk Dairy

Vegetable Proteins

- Legumes
- Nuts
- Protein powder
- Seeds

Fermented Foods

- Fermented vegetables
- Kimchi
- Raw sauerkraut
- Sheep or goat's milk kefir
- Sheep or goat's milk yogurt

Fruit

- Apples
- Avocados
- Berries
- Cherries
- Coconut
- Coconut water
- Grapefruit
- Kiwis
- Nectarines
- Oranges
- Pears
- Rhubarb
- Tangerines

Grains

- Brown Rice
- Millet
- Quinoa

Legumes

Beans of all types: black, black-eyed, navy, red, white, garbanzos, lentils

Vegetables

Artichokes
Asparagus
Beets
Black radishes
Bok choy
Broccoli and broccolini
Broccoli rabe
Brussels sprouts
Cabbage
Capers
Carrots (in cooking, not as a snack or side dish)
Cauliflower
Celery
Cucumbers
Dandelion Greens
Eggplant
Garlic
Kale
Kohlrabi
Jerusalem artichokes
Jicama
Lettuce (not iceberg)
Mushrooms
Onions
Potatoes
Radishes
Spinach
Squash
Tomatoes
Turnips

Nuts And Seeds

Nut butters
Nut flours
Nuts: Almonds, Brazil Nuts, Hazelnuts, Macadamia Nuts, Pecans, Pine Nuts, Walnuts
Seeds: Chia Seeds, Flaxseeds, Pumpkin Seeds, Sesame Seeds, Sunflower seeds

Oils

Avocado
Butter
Coconut Oil
Ghee
Extra Virgin Olive Oil

Spices

Cinnamon
Ginger
Turmeric

Of course, we are discovering new strains of probiotics and prebiotics all the time. "Microbiome Medicine," though based in ancient history is actually a new modality in healing. Science shows that this approach—removing toxins and bacterial enemies, adding foods rich in prebiotics, and introducing specific bacterial strains of probiotics—results in true healing, at the deepest level. My patients not only are relieved from their symptoms and illnesses, but find that they have renewed energy, optimism, and zest for life when they follow this protocol. Some feel better within a matter of days. I know that when you start this protocol, you will find many benefits as well!

I wish you all the best in your journey to good health.
Dr. Raphael Kellman

"We have a new model, a new way of understanding diseases. The key is understanding the bacteria and healing the microbiome. From that, we can heal countless numbers of people."
-Dr. Raphael Kellman, Founder of Microbiome Medicine

Kellman Center For Integrative and Functional Medicine
7 W. 45th Street, Suite 310
New York, NY 10036
212-717-1118
www.kellmancenter.com

Notes

PAGE 1

#1–National Institutes of Health, U.S. Department of Health and Human Services. *Opportunities and Challenges in Digestive Diseases Research: Recommendations of the National Commission on Digestive Diseases. Bethesda, MD: National Institutes of Health; 2009. NIH Publication 08-6514.*

#2–Changes in the nutrient content of the American diet: https://www.ncbi.nlm.nih.gov/pmc/articles/PMC3403271/

PAGE 2

#3–Revised Estimates for the Number of Human and Bacteria Cells in the Body: https://www.ncbi.nlm.nih.gov/pmc/articles/PMC4991899/

#4–Bacteria talk to each other and our cells in the same way, via molecules: https://www.sciencedaily.com/releases/2012/11/121106114241.htm

PAGE 3

#5–The inflammation theory of disease: The growing realization that chronic inflammation is crucial in many diseases opens new avenues for treatment: https://www.ncbi.nlm.nih.gov/pmc/articles/PMC3492709/

PAGE 10

#6–The Overuse of Antibiotics in Food Animals Threatens Public Health: https://consumersunion.org/news/the-overuse-of-antibiotics-in-food-animals-threatens-public-health-2/

PAGE 13

#7–Autoimmunity and the gut: https://www.ncbi.nlm.nih.gov/pmc/articles/PMC4036413/

#8 Berberine regulates neurite outgrowth through AMPK-dependent pathways by lowering energy status: https://www.ncbi.nlm.nih.gov/pubmed/25889370

PAGE 15

#9–Butyric acid in irritable bowel syndrome: https://www.ncbi.nlm.nih.gov/pmc/articles/PMC4027835/

PAGE 21

#10–Probiotics may help boost mood and cognitive function: https://www.health.harvard.edu/mind-and-mood/probiotics-may-help-boost-mood-and-cognitive-function

About the Author

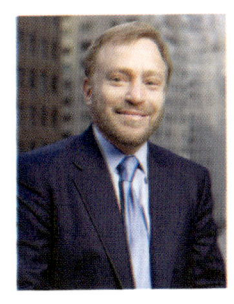

Raphael Kellman, MD, graduate of Albert Einstein College of Medicine, pioneered a groundbreaking new brand of medicine and healing, seamlessly integrating holistic and functional medicine with his visionary understanding of the world and nature, the root of who we are and its connection to health. Founder of "Microbiome Medicine," Dr. Kellman is a bestselling author, guest speaker and frequent lecturer. His most recent books are The Microbiome Breakthrough and The Microbiome Diet. As medical director of the Kellman Center in New York City, Dr. Kellman has treated tens of thousands of patients using his microbiome-centered approach to medicine. The Kellman Center specializes in thyroid disorders, gastro concerns, chronic fatigue, fibromyalgia, autism, anxiety, Lyme disease, cancer treatments, infertility, weight management, and unexplained malaise.